Hormones & Hair Loss

7 Natural Solutions to Help Menopausal Women Regrow Hair & Regain Their Confidence

---

Dr. Shawon Gullette, ND, I.A.T.

Hormones & Hair Loss: 7 Natural Solutions to Help Menopausal Women Regrow Hair & Regain Their Confidence

Copyright © 2017 by Dayton Trichology Hair Loss Control Center

All rights reserved. No part of this book may be reproduced or transmitted in any form or by any means without written permission from the author.

Printed in USA by Dayton Trichology Hair Loss Control Center

Dedication

This book is dedicated to my mother, Beverly Brown who has been my rock and my strength from day one! She insisted that I go to cosmetology school, which started a great career for me. Once I started Trichology School, she kept my daughter Mikashia Johnson every time I had to go away for clinical training, nights of studying, seminars, and speaking engagements.

Then, when I decided to pursue Naturopathic Medicine, she again, without hesitation stepped up to the plate and helped with my daughter. Currently, she is helping me with my grandson Caiyan. Filling in the gaps when I can't be there as I wish everyone that knows my mom knows that she is my number one supporter!

She keeps my business cards in her purse at all times and copies of my latest newspaper or magazine articles folded in her wallet, LOL.

Mom, you are my everything, and without you, I would not be the mother, Entrepreneur or woman I am today. Nor would I have a gratifying career that I have today. I love you Mom, for setting an excellent example for me and molding me into the woman, I am today and lastly but most importantly, encouraging me as a child to develop a relationship with Jehovah, God.

Table of Contents

Foreword 5

Introduction 8

Chapter 1: My Passion for Women's Hair Loss 18

Chapter 2: Silent No More 22

Chapter 3: The Anatomy of Hair............................... 30

Chapter 4: Hair Food... 45

Chapter 5: East & West.. 64

Chapter 6: It's in the Blood 69

Chapter 7: What About Other Options?.....................79

Chapter 8: Power of Twelve 87

Chapter 9: Why Seek Inspiration 95

Chapter 10: Estrogen Rich Recipes............................99

My Final Thoughts................................106

Foreword

As a mother of three daughters, I felt caught in an emotional war between my brother who decided to go bald and my mother who was experiencing extreme hair loss and thinning due to extreme hormone deficiency caused by menopause. I watched in horror as my mother, refused to leave her house for fear that someone at church or the supermarket would learn of her secret. Paralyzed with anxiety, I was helpless to aid my mother, a woman who had been such a source of strength to so many; fall victim to something so thin as the strains of hair.

It's amazing how society prepares young girls to appreciate their hair and commercials often-portrayed beautiful women with long flowing hair, full of body and silky smooth. However, society does not prepare women to deal with the psychological and emotional effects connected to hair loss. Instead, we're told, try a different shampoo, condition our hair more, or stop blow-drying our hair. All of which adds more stress and leaves us wondering, "Is there something wrong with me?"

For most men, hair loss begins as a receding hairline and is treated with topical solutions or hair replacement surgery.

Others like my brother opted to shave their heads. I remember several years ago after my brother decided to shave his head, and sent me a text that several women commented how sexy he looked. He also mentioned that if he had "known shaving his head would draw this type of attention; he would have shaved his head years ago."

While I wanted to celebrate my brother's excitement about the attention he was receiving, I felt torn because I could not shake the emotional discord I was feeling. I kept thinking, "why did women see my brother as sexy, while our mother was suffering in silence, afraid to face her friends and leave the house, it all seemed so unfair."

As I felt myself grasping for answers, I realized two things about those dealing with hair loss. First is the deep connection they have with their hair in the shaping of their identity and sex appeal. Second, the concerns they have about losing their hair. For some women, hair loss is more important than serious medical conditions, such as cancer and diabetes.

I know women who have refused chemotherapy because they could not imagine losing their hair, even if it meant saving their lives. Second, it's tough to understand the signs, cause and treatment of hair loss due to the significant amount of misinformation that exist on the Internet. How can you know if the information you read is accurate and based on real science? Thank heaven, I read Dr. Gullette's ND, book. I have found this book personally enlightening and a much-needed resource to help explain the root causes of hair loss for post-menopausal women. I appreciated the natural solutions offered that contributes to the regrowth of hair and more importantly, how it helps women to regain their confidence and vitality.

The book is written in such a way that it is entertaining and engaging with the use of relatable case studies. For me, I related to Lisa's story. Besides being entertaining, it's also medically accurate. Women desire to be informed about hair loss. However, they don't wish to read a textbook that is filled with medical terminology and jargon; this book provides the right balance. While I encourage readers to read the book from cover to cover, they will find the chapters informative, relevant, and pertinent to their situation.

I think Hair Loss: What's the Big Deal? Provides answers to questions that others and I have had related to hair loss, and options available. In my opinion, this book is necessary read and the best book I've read dedicated to post-menopausal hair loss.

Karen M.

Introduction

Since a child, I've dreamed of doing hair. Like most girls, I would spend hours combing and styling my dolls hair. As a teen, I attended John H. Patterson High school, which had a well-respected cosmetology program. I was excited to have my diploma and cosmetology license when I graduated in 1990.

In the 25 years that I have worked as a cosmetologist and hair stylist, I have had the opportunity to listen to the complaints of women dealing with how their hair loss has affected them emotionally. As a licensed cosmetologist, my training covered styling, and the chemical aspects of hair, but very little attention to Trichology, which is the scientific study of the hair, scalp disorders, and diseases. Trichology is discussed at length in chapter 4.

So when I had clients that experienced thinning hair and hair loss, my recourse; apply the leading brand of shampoos, conditioners, treatments, and hope for positive results. No matter what I used, the results were unpredictable; some worked, others didn't. It felt like a crap shoot! There had to be a better way; it was my desire to find it and share it with clients.

Not willing to give up, I began looking into other treatment methods, which led to my discovery of Trichology. My heart would break as I listened to women in tears, hit hard with a personal catastrophe that threatened their femininity because of thinning or loss of hair.

Perhaps one of the greatest discoveries I made during my journey to finding natural solutions to hormonally induced hair loss, was that I didn't have a full understanding between the correlation of the body and hair loss. A one-size-fits-all approach would not work; hair loss is personal, so treatments must also be personal, not generic. This quest for answers prompted me to obtain my Trichology certification from the International Association of Trichologist (I.A.T.).

Who Should Read this Book?

This book is written to encourage women suffering from hair loss due to hormonal issues caused by menopause. While the information in this book will benefit all women dealing with hair loss, it is written to help women understand that help is available, and this book provides seven natural solutions to help menopausal women regrow their hair and most importantly, regain their confidence.

It is crucial to understand that some issues may be beyond the skills and training of a cosmetologist, therefore, it would be best to refer clients to a certified Trichologist.

A Frantic Phone Call

One question that I am frequently asked at workshops and conferences, "Dr. Gullette ND, why are you so passionate about helping women with hair loss?" My answer is two-fold. First, as a woman, I can relate to my clients who are experiencing hair loss, because years ago, I had started losing my hair as a result of vitamin D and iron deficiencies. Second, I never will forget a frantic phone call I received back in 2005 while in school for Trichology, and working at the salon, when a client called in tears saying:

> "My name is Sarah, I have a 9-year-old daughter, Jessica whose hair is falling out in clumps when I wash it, comb it, brush it, even when I touch it, it just falls out."

I listened as Sarah drifted between weeping and the point of hysteria. At that moment, I was not a cosmetologist or hair stylist; I was a mother listening to another mother needing help. With my hand shaking from the eruptions of nerves; I scheduled them for an appointment, Thursday morning 9 a.m., deep inside, I kept trying to convince myself everything was fine and to focus on my training. I remember thinking, "Shawon, it's okay, don't get emotional, it's no big deal."

Thursday was two days away; I tried to be professional at work, and for the most part, I was. The drive to and from work was the hardest. Heading to work, my thoughts remained captured by images of this precious little girl losing her hair and kids laughing at her, because kids at that age can be unintentionally cruel. When I left work, I thought about my own my daughter and what I would do if she faced similar challenges?

The drive to the salon on Thursday filled my body with anxiety as a contemplated what I would see once I arrived at the shop. Hands shaking, mouth dry and heart beating as if someone was playing the drums on my chest, I open the door, and Sarah was sitting there with Jessica waiting. They had arrived ten minutes early. Jessica was oblivious to what was going on in the salon, there she was, a beautiful, bright-eyed little girl, sitting in the chair with hair pulled back in a big bushy ponytail playing with her doll. In some ways, Jessica reminded me of myself playing with the hair on her doll.

Taking a deep breath, I approached Sarah and introduced myself, voice a bit scratchy, 'Hello, my name is Shawon." Once introduced, I took both Sarah and Jessica to the private consultation room, putting a robe around her and I was shocked when after releasing the rubber band that held her ponytail together noticed 3 to 4 circular patches missing from her head. Some were the size of lemons, while other spots resembled the size of a small orange.

During my training, we had covered this type of hair loss (alopecia arearta) and now; I saw it first-hand, not in an adult, but a little girl. I knew I had to keep it together because Sarah needed me to be a source of strength, compassion, and assure her that there was a treatment or cure to reverse her baby's hair loss; the sad reality, there was no treatment or cure for her daughter's hair loss.

There we stood, as the tears swelled in the corner of Sarah's eyes and one single tear created a thin track down the cheek of her face. We stood in my consultation office, knowing that we were connected forever by a little girl's loss of hair. No amount of education or training can prepare for the harsh realities of life when it involves children. I have witnessed strong men reduced to emotional rubble at the sight of an injured or terminally ill child.

At the request of Sarah, I applied some shampoo and hair conditioner to Jessica's hair; once I started washing her hair, it quickly turned into a tangled web that looked like a matted black cotton ball. There I stood, looking at Sarah and wondering if I should have washed her hair or referred her to someone else? I had to do something, I pulled out my shears and agonized if my only solution at this point was to cut Jessica's hair off or try something else?

All I could think about was my daughter, and as a mother, the terror she must be experiencing in that moment. I thought about how did this happen, why had fate dealt her such an unwelcome blow? I didn't know all of the answers, but I knew I had to make a decision.

Before deciding my course of action, I thought about how her life from that day forward would change, and how my life and Sarah's life would be transformed that day.

I pulled out my shears and "snip" the big bushy ponytail that had morphed into a cotton ball laid silently at my feet, it was forever gone. Gone were the memories that helped shaped this precious little soul, gone were the thoughts and compliments that she'd received, all that remained was a close cut head that from back made her unrecognizable as the girl who entered the salon a few minutes prior. In an agonizing voice, her mother asked, "why is my baby's hair falling out?"

In response, I explained that Jessica's spotty hair loss is typical of a condition known as *alopecia areata,* which is an autoimmune disease. Despite the social stigma, this has on children; it is actually common. Her hair loss is due to her body cells fighting against and destroying its own tissue. In about 1 to 2% of cases, it can spread to the entire scalp (alopecia totalis) or the entire body (alopecia universalis).

What's happening in Jessica's body is that her T cell lymphocytes (white blood cells) cluster around her affected follicles, causing it to become inflamed and fall out. Alopecia areata most often affects the scalp, but can show on any part of the body with hair.

It was important for me to let Sarah know that alopecia areata is not contagious, and research supports the notion that heredity could be a factor.

My experience with little nine-year-old Jessica and women of all ages became my motivation to become a certified Trichologist. Having this certification, the first in Ohio for many years, provided me the skills and training needed to treat diseases and disorders of the hair and scalp. I was knowledgeable   about virtually every type of hair loss and the reasons from a clinical viewpoint. My focused became hair loss and its connection to hormones, especially the endocrine system.

Realizing that many of the causes connected to hair loss were results of poor health and nutrition, I again set out on a journey to help my clients, especially women losing their hair due to the effects of menopause. I decided to return to school and studied Naturopathic Medicine in order to help me understand the correlation between the body, its systems and a holistic approach to treatment.

What's the Big Deal

Some may feel that the issue of hair loss is not a big deal. In their mind, hair loss is about vanity and misplaced priorities. They fail to recognize that over 30 million women are suffering from hair loss. There are many reasons for this widespread incidence. Although most of these women will never completely lose all their hair, they may experience thinning or diffuse hair loss (all over the head).

As humans, we have been a concern with our appearance dating back to antiquity. In fact, during ancient times, there were some interesting discoveries. For example, eunuchs: males without genitals due to castration battle, accidents, punishment or while in their youth never went bald. This was the first indication that hormones (testosterone) had something to do with hair loss.

Crown of Glory

In many cultures, like in the United States, hair is considered a woman's "Crown of Glory" and is very much associated with her beauty and status in society. Hair loss in women can be devastating; it affects their self-esteem, confidence, work ethic, and can cause undue stress on the body. Here are several facts about hair loss:

- Approximately 30 million women (one in four) experience hereditary female hair loss or baldness.

- 40% of women never expected to face the challenge of hair loss or baldness

- 50% of women experience hair loss by middle age

Typically, your hair is at its thickest at age 20. After 20, your hair gradually begins to thin, shedding more than the usual 40-100 hairs each day. Fine hair is both a precursor for and consequence of hair thinning. Women who experience hair loss have a disproportionately high rate of fine hair before they start losing their hair.

Here is the Big Deal

Hair loss in women becomes an appearance issue, and it can also be the cause of severe emotional stress for most women. A recent study reported that women have a difficult time confronting hair loss:

- Female study participants under age 50 reported feeling a "severe emotional blow."
- 29% admitted feeling scared
- 47% said they were embarrassed
- 15% felt unattractive
- 28% experienced paranoia

As a Doctor of Naturopathic Medicine, I look beyond symptoms to the root causes of hair loss in women. I always tell my patients:

"Your hair is an indication of what's going on in the body."

Dr. Shawon Gullette ND, I.A.T.

1

My Passion for Women's Hair Loss

Sometimes, it is hard for me to believe that I have been in the hair business for over twenty-five years. Thomas Edison once said, "I have never worked a day in my life, it has all been fun." Reflecting on this quote reminds me that I have not worked a day in my adult life. This comment simply implies that I truly enjoy the work that I do, and it is hard to consider it work; despite some days being more challenging than others, overall, what I do is a calling and fulfillment of my purpose in life.

Drawn to the field of hair care as a young child and later dedicating my life to work with women dealing with issues related to hair loss in general. Since taking my first cosmetology course in high school, I have been fascinated with hair science. From its molecular structure and chemical components, hair has always been interesting to me; especially how hair grows, its various textures.

When I see a client in my clinic and hear their stories and depiction of how they feel and how society has treated them because of losing their hair; it has stuck with me. Here is the truth, despite your age, race, income, or social class, hair loss is an issue that matters to over 30 million women in this country. Why does it matter so much? It matters because hair speaks to the very meaning of beauty and acceptance for women and when they lose their hair, it affects their sense of being human. I have heard women refer to themselves as monsters, ugly, sexually undesirable sexually and emotionally paralyzed.

The benefits of being a certified Trichologist is that I understand many aspects of my client's experiences and how best to develop a unique and personal treatment plan specific to the individual. On occasions, I will see clients with similar hair and scalp conditions, and symptoms, but due to their lifestyle differences, leave with two very different treatment plans. I don't utilize any generic approaches or a 'one-size-fits-all template; in my clinic, each client is treated as an individual with specific needs, which requires a personalized plan of treatment and aftercare follow-up visits.

Second, I am a naturopathic doctor (ND) who treats clients from a holistic perspective. I work to help clients make lifestyle changes that can benefit them; my specialty is working with menopausal women, and there have been some great moments, too many to list. It gives me great joy to see clients regain their confidence and self-esteem after regrowing their hair and coming to terms with the reality that their hair alone did not define who they were as a person. In many ways, this is the reason I became an ND to apply my knowledge of hair and natural cures and treatments to hair loss.

Currently, my goal has shifted to reaching a larger audience through education and that is why I decided to write a book. Individually, I can only reach so many people, however, through my educational resources, which include webinars, workshops, video blog and publications; I can affect a greater number of people searching for naturopathic solutions to hair loss due to menopause.

My greatest hope is to inspire another generation of Trichologist to adapt a holistic approach to treating hair. I know as an industry, we have a lot of work to do in bringing awareness to hair loss, and its affects on the psyche. To some, my goals may seem too lofty; nevertheless, I know it will materialize someday. I just have to continue to keep the faith and press forward, enjoying the journey along the way. As I stated before, I'm having too much fun to consider what I do as work; it's my calling and purpose in life.

In the next chapter, we will meet two extraordinary women, Maggie and Jill as they share their remarkable stories of dealing with hair loss. I share their remarkable stories of strength and courage to demonstrate the power of the human spirit and the importance of seeking help, so that no woman will suffer in silence due to feeling shame because of their hair loss.

2

Silent No More

Maggie's Story

I'm 57 years old from the North Eastern part of the United State. I've been married for close to thirty years, and we have four beautiful grown children. My husband, Chuck is a larger than life big guy with a teddy bear heart. He is an excellent man and has been emotionally supportive of my depression concerning my hair loss.

Several months ago, I asked him to accompany me to a hair specialty shop to pick out a wig. I was so excited to have Chuck with me that day. We stopped at our favorite restaurant for lunch and held hands as we walked a few blocks to the specialty shop which was in walking distance. Chuck, made me feel alive again, it had been several months since we had been on a date. Not that he didn't try to get me out of the house, I was too embarrassed to go and felt that everyone's eyes were fixed on me. I knew it was in my head, but it felt real to me.

As we entered the store, Chuck sat down in a chair and started reading a magazine; it must have been a seating area for men because two other men were also reading magazines with the occasional glance to see if their partner was in the checkout aisle. After twenty minutes, a record for me, I found the perfect wig, I motioned for Chuck to come and see my purchase and to approve the $798 price tag.

Once he saw the price, he softly asked if this would make me happy and get back to my old self? I looked into his eyes and responded, "I feel like I did when we first got married, plus, this is real Brazillian hair." "In that case, it's worth the price." He replied. Chuck didn't say much walking back to the car. Then he said, "now that you bought your hair, I won't have to hear you complain about your hair and not being able to hang out with our friends, right?"

My excitement and prospect of feeling attractive again caused Chuck's words to fall on deaf ears. As the days turned to weeks, I noticed that the excitement and joy I once felt faded into feelings of self-doubt and depression. "I am so stupid," I thought. It's been three months since my purchase, and I was not back to my regular self, I was worse than before. Before I refused to look at myself in the mirror. Not anymore, I felt arrested by its grip, standing their self-loathing at what lies beneath my wig and hating myself for spending so much money on a pipe dream. Besides, every morning after my shower; large strands of hair are left in the tub, it's beyond disgusting.

The other night, Chuck tried to be intimate with me and accidently pulled off my scarf; immediately I snapped at him and accused him of mocking me. I even went to far as to accused him of not loving me and only caring about satisfying himself. Since then, Chuck has withdrawn into a shell, barely talking to me and sleeping near the edge of the bed.

I hate what my hair loss has turned me into lately. As for my expensive wig, it has been retired to the box in my closet. I'm tired of feeling depressed during the day, and crying myself to sleep at night.

A part of me believes that Chuck wanted to believe that buying the wig would fix my emotional issues. He doesn't realize I'm dying inside, despite the fact at times I just grin and bear it. Chuck is my rock, and I don't know how to explain what's going on with me emotionally because I don't understand it. I was told by my sister-in-law to contact Dr.

Gullette ND, so I hope she can tell me what's going on in my body.

My Assessment of Maggie
When examining Maggie's case, her hair loss may be caused by hormones depletion. Hormones regulate the activity of cells and tissues in various organs of the body. The balance of hormones produced by your body is essential to good health and a feeling of well-being.

Jill's Story

Turning 49 is not what I thought it would be. That's when I first noticed my brush full of hair. I thought maybe it was caused by brushing too hard or having dry, brittle hair. I tried everything and nothing worked. I know this sounds vain and shallow, but if I had to choose between receiving a million dollars in cash or keeping a full head of hair; I think, no I know that I would want to keep my hair.

Eight months ago, two events happened. First I started going through the change, menopause, and second, I found out from my supervisor Tom, that my position and the entire division was being relocated to Mexico." I thought he was joking! How could this be happening? At that moment I felt my breath leave my body and I stood there emotionless as a piece of marble in shock at the news.

Shipped overseas to Mexico, what about my home, kids, and my life here in the states? Tom tried to console me by saying, 'Jill, you would keep the same pay and they would help with selling your home and find you an apartment in Mexico but they need your decision in six weeks."

Six weeks to try to grapple with this news was not fair. I had been with the company for almost twenty-three years and never thought I would have to choose between relocating to another country to keep my job or resign and face the uncertainty of the job market.

Two weeks later, I noticed small amounts of my hair falling out, but I was not that concerned because I just figured it was the new shampoo I was using which made my hair a little dryer than other shampoos. I switched back to my regular shampoo, and for about a month, things seemed to be fine, until it was two weeks before I had to respond and that whole day I was a mess.

I couldn't sleep, eat, or think. I even forgot that I left eggs on the stove until the smoke detector sounded and scared me to death. I walked into the kitchen, and the pot was smoking from the scorched eggs which resembled two pieces of burnt charcoal. I turned off the stove and placed the pot in the sink, with the faucet on; watching as the water popped and pot buckle from the cold water. The pot was trash; I opened the window to allow the smoke to escape the kitchen.

Smelling the stench of burnt eggs made me sick, and I desperately needed a shower. In the shower, I felt as if my body was on fire from stress, I washed my hair and afterward while drying it; I fell to my knees when I pulled out two patches of my hair which left behind two small bald spots near the back of my neck. What was happening to me? The following day, I visited my salon, and the stylist sold me a bottle of expensive shampoo and conditioner. I tried it for several days, and each time I dried my hair, I noticed my hair continued to fall out.

The day I made my decision to resign my position was the hardest thing I ever had to do. I gave Tom my letter of resignation and explained that I could not leave my family and life behind to go to a country I didn't know. Tom understood and explained that I would receive a severance package that included three months of pay and I would continue to keep my health benefits for six months. Appreciative of the opportunity given me over the years, I packed twenty-two years of my work experience into a small white box and walked out the door.

I sat in my car for thirty minutes and wept. I prayed, "God, what am I to do now?" I had no job, no connections and no answers to why my hair was falling out. I scheduled an appointment to see a dermatologist and the treatments prescribed helped to reduce the amount of hair loss, but didn't stop my hair from falling out.

I don't know if my menopause or the stress of my job is causing my hair to fall out. That's when a friend suggested I visit Dr. Gullette's ND, clinic. I scheduled an appointment, hoping she can help me understand what's going on and how to reverse my hair loss.

<u>My Assessment of Jill</u>
Often, there is a primary diagnosis which can be attributed to menopause, however; stress can cause Jill's adrenal glands which are the "stress" glands of the body; stress increases the production of hormones from the adrenal cortex and the medulla. [1]

In the upcoming chapter I will discuss the anatomy of your hair to give you an understanding of the cycle of hair growth.

---

[1]https://www.ncbi.nlm.nih.gov/pmc/articles/PMC4997656/

Key Point #1

"Understanding hair loss is the beginning of finding the right treatment options."

3

The Anatomy of Hair

While this book is about hair loss, caused by hormone depletion or dominance (estrogen) in postmenopausal women, it is essential that I discuss the natural growth cycle of human hair. Every day, on average, we shed between fifty to hundred hair follicles, which is normal.

Hair is the fastest growing tissue of the body, made up of proteins called keratins. Every strand of hair has three layers: the inner layer or medulla (only present in thick hairs); the middle layer or cortex, which determines the strength, texture, and color of hair; and the cuticle, which protects the cortex. Each strand of hair on our heads is a complex weaving of proteins in the hair follicle. Hair follicles are tiny organs consisting of living cells, which receive nutrients from the blood supply beneath the skin.

Our hair goes through three unique stages, which are:

- Anagen Stage
- Catagen Stage
- Telogen Stage

First, is the Anagen Stage, or "growing" stage of a hair follicle. As a miniaturized hair follicle, the hair begins to grow; when this happens, it starts to extend deep into the skin creating a new hair bulb. The hair bulb is a collection of specialized dermal papilla cells, which forms a new hair shaft. In essence, the new hair growth helps to "push" out the old hair from the follicle. This new hair extends from the surface of the skin as either curly or straight at an average rate of one-half inch per month for scalp hairs. Color variations may range from brown, red, blonde, or gray.

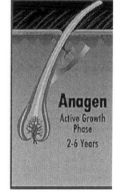

Second, the hair begins to regress or stop growing, causing the hair follicle to shrink. This "regression" is known as the Catagen Stage. During this part of the hair cycle, the bottom portion of the hair follicle disintegrates, requiring fewer nutrients from the blood supply. It is natural for follicles to atrophy and hair to

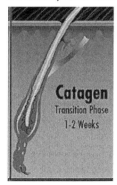

fall out. As this continues, the base of the hair bulb structure disappears, and dermal papilla cells separate from the base of the follicle. When the miniaturized hair follicle loses its "grip" on the hair shaft, any daily grooming activities such as bathing might result in shedding the hair shaft. This stage typically lasts two to three weeks.

The final stage is when the hair follicle stops shrinking, and enters a "resting" stage, referred to as the Telogen Stage lasting about ninety days. In this stage, the hair follicle is dormant and, shed hairs end up on your pillow, clothing, and brushes or in the tub after shampooing your hair. When this cycle ends, it begins to repeat the cycle again. [2]

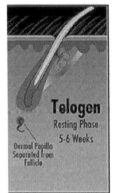

The range of hair loss may be large and persistent, bald patches, loss of scalp hair (alopecia totalis) and in severe cases, loss of all body hair which may persist for short or long periods (alopecia universalis). Regardless of type, hair regrowth is possible because the issue rests with inflammation within the bulb structure, which regenerates during the hair growth cycle.

---

[2] https://www.ncbi.nlm.nih.gov/pmc/articles/PMC4606321/

According to research conducted by The National Alopecia Areata Foundation, about two percent of the US population at some point in their lives will suffer some form of alopecia. While non-life threatening, alopecia areata affects (bald spots) can have a profound psychological impact on those affected especially children.

It is vital then to take care of the scalp and body to perpetuate hair growth and maintenance. Expensive treatments that claim to treat the visible hair and nourish it, are usually no more than bogus claims made to sell products. If for no other reason, it's important to consult a certified Trichologist trained in the study of hair and scalp issues. You may be asking yourself, 'What is Trichology?"

What is Trichology?

Trichology is the medical term for the study of the hair (and scalp) and all problems related to them. A 'Trichologist' is someone who specializes in hair loss problems such as baldness, hair breakage, and itchy/flaking scalp. He or she will also treat all forms of alopecia.

A Trichologist is someone you may wish to consult to do a complete examination of your hair and scalp. The condition of your hair is an indicator of your general health. Hair that is dull and lifeless can suggest a stressed, unhealthy lifestyle whereas hair that is full and shiny may be a sign of being healthy. This is one of the several factors considered when deciding upon suitable treatment options.

If he or she feels that there is an underlying medical cause, then he/she will advise you to visit your medical doctor. You do not have to have a hair problem to consult a Trichologist: many people choose to do so because they want advice on keeping their hair and scalp in tip-top condition and reduce the risk of hair loss. Prevention is better than cure and doing this can save you time and money in the long term.

The client may complain of sudden excessive hair loss from all over the scalp, a bald patch that has suddenly appeared, or itching and excessive scaling of the scalp. A microscopic examination of the hair might be required to aid in the diagnosis of the problem. Then the Trichologist would determine if treatment is necessary which might consist of the application of a particular cream or lotion to the scalp or the use of nutritional therapy.

Within the field of hair loss, there are two scales that Trichologist and Dermatologist use to measure hair thinning, the Savin and Ludwig scale. Both scales are identical, except that the Savin Scale measures overall thinning. There are eight-crown density images, which indicate the ranges from no hair loss to severe hair loss.

In the first image, (labeled I-1) the central parting of along the scalp shows no hair loss. Images 2 to 4 (labeled I-2, I-3, and I-4) shows the width of the parting along the scalp progressively widening which indicates the thinning of the hair.

The images labeled II-1 and II-2 show diffuse thinning of the hair over the top of the scalp. The image labeled III shows a woman with extensive diffuse hair loss on top of the scalp, with some surviving hair.

The image labeled "advanced" is a woman with extensive hair loss with little to no surviving hair in the affected area. A small percentage of women reach this stage and when they do, it is most likely caused by abnormally excessive androgen hormone production.

The last image is "frontally accentuated" where there is more hair loss near the front and center of the scalp instead of the top middle part of the scalp.

Pictured below is the popular Savin scale: [3]

---

[3] http://www.themeter.net/ludwig_e.htm

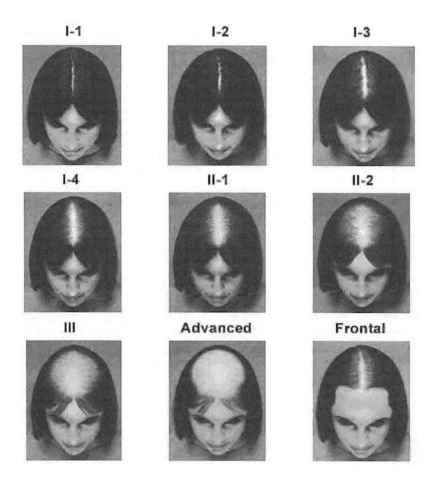

The Ludwig Classification divides female pattern baldness (androgenetic into 1 of 3 grades on the scale. Classification is essential to helping you understand three key factors used in the diagnosis and treatment of your hair loss: (1) Degree of hair already lost, (b) potential for future hair loss, (c) best treatment options. Here are the various grades:

Grade I. Hair loss is **mild**. Most will have difficulty noticing that hair loss, as the frontal hairline remains relatively
unaffected. It will become noticeable when the hair is parted down the center of the scalp and more of the scalp is exposed over time.

Grade II. Moderate hair loss is when women begin to notice thinning, shedding, and a general decrease in hair thickness and volume, the center part continues to widen.

Grade III. Extreme hair loss in which hair become very fine and thin, making it difficult to camouflage the scalp, making it visible to the naked eye.

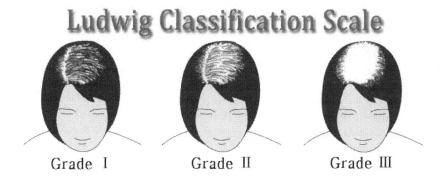

Lifestyle & Hair Loss

When you are experiencing hair loss, it could be an indication that there is something wrong internally in the body. Improper nutrition, unhealthy lifestyles, and crash diets are some of the culprits that can contribute to hair loss. Hair loss cannot be corrected until you make a conscience effort to make changes to your health and well-being. For hair to grow healthy there needs to be adequate nutrition and energy at the hair follicle. Since the hair follicle is not a tissue that is essential to the body, it is the last tissue to receive its energy supply. Also, the hair follicle is the first tissue to have its energy supply reduced if there are other areas in the body that have a shortage of energy.

One of the biggest lifestyle changes you can make is eliminating or reducing your sugar consumption. Research has shown that sugar can lead to a hormone imbalance in the body. Herbal teas can increase estrogen levels and offer you relief from the symptoms associated with menopause or premenstrual syndrome without affecting your estrogen levels. You should steep the herbs for at least five minutes in hot water. A good tea is Red clover, which has isoflavones and may reduce the symptoms of menopause or premenstrual syndrome.

Most nutritional deficiencies cause temporary hair loss that is corrected, once you resolve the disturbance within the body. A healthy diet, and happier lifestyles and the use of supplements can influence optimal hair growth. If you ignore the signs of your hair loss and the disturbance is prolonged, it can lead to permanent hair loss, or speed up a predisposed hair loss condition.

Hair, Scalp Diseases & Disorders

There are a variety of hair and scalp diseases and disorders, some of which are very common, while others are more severe and rare. Here I discuss some of the common hair and scalp diseases.

Alopecia Areata which affects 1.7 percent of the world population, including 4.7 million people in the United States. There is no known cause for alopecia areata and therefore no known cure. However, David Salinger noted that "cortisones will worsen genetic hair loss, but can be of a benefit with autoimmune problems such as alopecia areata and scarring alopecia."

The disease usually hits before age 20 and does not seem to favor one particular gender or culture. Hair loss with alopecia areata comes in stages, with hair returning and falling out in phases.

In 2010, a genome-wide association study examined 129 single nucleotide polymorphism associated with alopecia areata. The genes controlled the proliferation of regulatory T cells, cytotoxic T lymphocyte-associated antigen 4, interleukin-2, interleukin-2 receptor A. Two specific genes: PRDX5 and STX17, are located in the hair follicle. [4] Here are a few terms to know:

- Alopecia areata monolocularis which baldness in one spot on the head. Alopecia areata multilocularis refers to multiple areas of hair loss.
- Alopecia Ophiasis is hair loss resembling a wave at the circumference of the head.
- Alopecia barbae which tend to be limited to the beard area.
- When all the hair is loss on the scalp is called Alopecia areata totalis.
- In some cases, all of the body's hair is gone, including pubic hair is known as alopecia universalis.

Seborrhea is the form of the disease where oiliness only occurs without redness and scaling. The disease commonly occurs in infants, middle-aged people, and the elderly, and commonly known in infants as cradle cap. The disease has

---

[4] https://www.naaf.org/advance-research/clinical-research

no cure, yet in infants, it usually disappears in time. With adults, the condition may persist with varying degrees of severity.

Seborrheic Dermatitis, an advanced form of seborrhea, is a non-contagious skin disease that causes excessive oiliness of the skin, most commonly in the scalp, caused by overproduction of sebum, and yeast (fungus) called malassezia. This is caused from oil secretion on the skin produced by the body to lubricate the skin where hair follicles are present. [5]

Psoriasis is an immune-mediated disorder that affects different areas and functions of the body. It is non-contagious, and one of the areas of the body it can affect is the scalp. It usually appears as patches of raised red skin accompanied by burning and itching. [6] Several contributing factors thought to contribute to the outbreak of psoriasis, including emotional stress, certain infections, toxemia, the thinning of the intestinal walls and adverse reactions to certain drugs.

At least half of people who have psoriasis have scalp psoriasis. Like seborrhea, scalp psoriasis left untreated can

[5] http://www.mayoclinic.org/diseases-conditions/seborrheic-dermatitis/basics/causes/con-20031872
[6] http://www.webmd.com/skin-problems-and-treatments/psoriasis/research#1

cause hair loss. Fortunately, you can treat it with a variety of topical creams and shampoos containing tar and salicylic acid. It is vital not to scratch the scalp and pick at the scabs that psoriasis causes, as this could damage the hair follicles in the dermis and cause permanent hair loss. As long as the follicles are not damaged, hair loss caused by this malady is usually temporary, and hair will grow back once the condition clears.

Eczema is another non-contagious skin disease that mimics psoriasis very closely. Eczema produces scales, reddened inflamed skin that periodically ooze and the familiar itch that is of supreme annoyance to those that suffer with it. These are however two different diseases that usually require different treatments. However, there are certain treatments that work for psoriasis that work for eczema also.

Eczema causes extreme buildup and sores on the scalp and can cause severe scarring. The buildup caused by eczema can cause temporary hair loss; however, the scarring that can occur if scratched can cause permanent damage to the hair follicle.

Chemotherapy treatments are found to cause skin sensitivity and to extremely irritating to the scalp. For this reason, I felt it important to mention in this section because one of the major side effects of this treatment is that it also destroys cells that promote the growth of hair and nails. Fortunately, hair normally returns within six months to a year after treatments cease. Patients have found that hair re-grown after chemotherapy is finer in texture and lighter in color at first.

These usually temporary conditions improve with time. Those recovering from chemotherapy should avoid chemical processes such as perms, relaxers, bleaching and coloring of the hair until it grows at least three inches and not until at least one year after the last treatment.

Key Point #2

"Nutritional deficiencies that cause temporary hair loss can be corrected once you resolve the disturbance within the body."

4

Hair Foods

In the previous chapters, I was speaking as a Trichologist and Cosmetologist with over 25 years of experience. In the next two chapters, I will be addressing you from a Naturopathic medicine perspective. One of the best ways to maintain your health is through a healthy diet and exercise regimen.

Although certain factors contribute to hair loss, we must keep in mind that hair is part of the complete biological system of the human body. Dysfunctions in one part of the system can contribute to dysfunctions in other parts; causing chain reactions to occur when one part of the body malfunctions.

Defining a healthy diet when it comes to preventing hair loss is complex. Principally, the main vitamins, minerals, and nutrients known to promote and maintain healthy hair are vitamin A, all B vitamins-particularly vitamins B-6 and B-12, folic acid, biotin, vitamin C, vitamin E, copper, iron, zinc, iodine, protein of course, silica, essential fatty acids (EFA's, formerly known as vitamin F) and last but not least, water.

The best way to maintain a healthy vitamin and mineral intake is a good diet. It is not necessary or advisable to go out and buy a bunch of over-the-counter vitamin supplements to achieve your suggested nutritional levels. In fact, many over-the-counter vitamins are chemically processed and not completely absorbed into your system. It is also easy to overdose with over the counter vitamins particularly when taking fat-soluble vitamins and minerals supplements, causing toxicity and adverse reactions.

The likelihood of doing this is far less with food; therefore, it is always best to obtain the bulk of your vitamin and mineral requirements from whole foods. I will discuss each vitamin and mineral to give you a better understanding of how nutrition is vital to healthy hair and may help with hair regrowth.

Vitamin A is a key component to developing healthy cells and tissues in the body, including hair. Additionally, it works with silica and zinc to prevent drying and clogging of the sebaceous glands, the glands vital to producing sebum, which is an important lubricant for the hair follicle. Vitamin A deficiencies commonly cause thickening of the scalp, dry hair, and dandruff.

Air pollution, smoking, extremely bright light, certain cholesterol-lowering drugs, laxatives, and aspirin are some well-known vitamin A inhibitors. Liver, fish oil, eggs, fortified milk, and red, yellow, and orange vegetables are good sources of vitamin A, as are some dark green leafy vegetables like spinach.

Be particularly careful if you take vitamin A supplements, as vitamin A is fat-soluble, allowing the body to store it and making it easy to overdose. Vitamin A overdoses can cause excessively dry skin and inflamed hair follicles, and in some cases ironically can cause hair loss. If you choose to take supplements of this vitamin, consult with a specialist first. As mentioned above, the likelihood of overdosing by achieving your vitamin A intake by food sources is almost nil, so it is best to attempt to achieve this at all costs.

B-vitamins work interdependently, and therefore all levels of B vitamins need to be sufficient to maintain proper health. Vitamins B-6, folic acid, biotin, and Vitamin B-12 are all key components in maintaining healthy hemoglobin levels in the blood, which is the iron-containing portion of red-blood cells. Hemoglobin's primary function is to carry oxygen from the lungs to the tissues of the body, so if these vitamins were deficient in one's body, then hair and skin would indeed suffer.

Fortunately, some of the tastiest foods contain these vitamins. Vitamin B-6 is in protein-rich foods, which is excellent because the body needs a sufficient amount of protein to maintain hair growth as well. Liver, chicken, fish, pork, kidney, and soybeans are good sources of B-6 and are relatively low in fat when they are not fried.

Folic acid is found in whole grains, cereals, nuts, green leafy vegetables, orange juice, brewer's yeast, wheat germ, and liver again. Meat, fish, poultry, eggs, and other dairy products meanwhile provide healthy amounts of B-12. Biotin deficiencies are rare unless there is a severe case of malnutrition or a serious intestinal disorder since a healthy gut produces biotin through good bacteria found there.

Note: if you have a known intestinal disorder and are plagued by hair loss, ask your doctor about biotin deficiencies and possible solutions.

Vitamin C is responsible for the development of healthy collagen, which is necessary to hold body tissues together. A vitamin C deficiency can cause split ends and hair breakage, yet this is easily reversible with an increase to normal vitamin C levels. Vitamin C is found in foods such as fresh peppers, citrus fruits, melons berries, potatoes, tomatoes, and dark green leafy vegetables.

Vitamin E is necessary to provide good blood circulation to the scalp by increasing the uptake of oxygen. Vitamin E is derived from foods such as green leafy vegetables, nuts, grains, vegetable oils, and most ready-to-eat cereals. Vitamin E deficiencies are rare in people in North America and Europe. In the rare cases of vitamin E deficiency, usually caused by the inability to absorb oils and fats, dietary supplements are available.

Omega-3 and Omega-6 fatty acid. A research study published in the Journal of Cosmetic Dermatology indicated that the supplementation of omega-3 and omega-6 fatty acids, plus antioxidants, prevented hair loss in the women tested and improved the thickness of their hair. The use of omega-3 and omega-6 showed a positive effect on the overall scalp coverage through a reduced telogen percentage, hair thickness, reduced miniaturized hair ratio and the increased perceived diameter after 6 months of daily intake. [7]

Copper is a trace mineral that is also necessary for the production of hemoglobin. Hemoglobin, as mentioned earlier, is vital to the process of carrying oxygen to tissues such as the hair, and obviously hair is alive cannot grow without proper oxygen, yet it does not breathe as other components of our body do because the oxygen must get to the shaft of the hair. Good sources of copper are liver again, seafood, nuts, and seeds.

Sulphur, according to a research study conducted by doctors Jacob and Lawrence in their book "The Miracle of MSM" noted that sulfur is nature's 'beauty mineral' for keeping the hair healthy and the complexion youthful." More specific, MSM sulfur (methyl-sulphonyl-methane) is a white, odorless, water-soluble element found in milk, eggs, onions, garlic, asparagus and broccoli. The mineral study, published in Total Health Magazine was shown to increased hair growth while conducting a placebo-controlled trial over the course of six weeks. Thirty percent of the subjects

---

[7] Effect of a nutritional supplement on hair loss in women. J Cosmet Dermatol, 14: 76–82. doi:10.1111/jocd.12127

showed improvement in hair brilliance, while none of the subjects on placebo showed such an improvement.

Another key mineral vital in the production of hemoglobin is iron. **Iron** is found in two forms, heme, and non-heme; heme iron is much easier to absorb into the system. This is where the problem lies. Of course, most people know that red meat is a good source of iron. However, red meat is non-heme iron and is difficult for the body to absorb, as are many iron supplements. Good heme iron sources are green leafy vegetables, kidney beans, and bran. Additionally, one can increase the absorption of non-heme iron into the body by consuming non-heme food sources and vitamin C sources in the same meal.

Zinc is another vital component to healthy hair, being that it is responsible for cell production, tissue growth and repair, and the maintenance of the oil-secreting glands of the scalp. It also plays a large role in protein synthesis and collagen formation. For this reason, zinc is important for both hair maintenance and dandruff prevention.

Most Americans are deficient in zinc. Most foods of animal origin, particularly seafood, contain good amounts of zinc; oysters are particularly rich in zinc. Zinc is also found in eggs and milk, although in much smaller amounts. Zinc from sources such as nuts, legumes, and natural grains is of a different type than those found in animal sources and is not easily used by the body, although oats are a good source of zinc that is readily used by the body.

Protein in most of the animal source foods, particularly meats, fish, milk, cheese, eggs, and yogurt. There is no need for a person eating the average Western diet to eat additional protein. Too much protein will not improve hair growth and may cause other health problems.

A challenge for vegans is to maintain healthy levels of protein, being that complete proteins containing all nine essential amino acids necessary are found mostly in animal sources. Legumes, seeds, nuts, grains, and vegetables do not contain the same form of protein necessary for a healthy body.

There is only one common non-meat source of complete protein, and that is the soybean. Soybeans, a texturized vegetable protein (TVP) can become a variety of different dishes. Additionally, one may eat from a wide variety of vegetable sources to obtain all the essential amino acids.

Iodine is vital to the growth of hair. Sheep farmers long ago discovered that vegetation void of iodine due to the iodine-depleted soil would adversely affect the growth of wool in sheep. Likewise, our hair needs iodine to grow, added synthetically to table salt; in this form, it is poorly absorbed into the body and can cause iodine overload.

Too much iodine in the body can adversely affect the thyroid. It is best to use non-iodized salt and retrieve your iodine from natural food sources. These include seaweed, salmon, seafood, lima beans, molasses, eggs, potatoes with the skin on, watercress and garlic.

One of the most difficult nutrients vital to hair growth to get in one's diet is the trace mineral silica. Silica is a form of silicon and is the second most abundant element in the earth's crust, second only to oxygen. The Earth provides everything we need for health, and with silicon being so abundant, it would seem that there would never be a problem with silica deficiency.

Unfortunately, trace minerals are rare in Western diets because chemical treatments deplete our soil food has lost trace minerals. Even most of the foods in our supermarkets are processed. Silica is vital to the strength of hair, and although it will not necessarily stop hair from falling out from the follicle, it will stop hair breakage. It works by stimulating the cell metabolism and formation, which slows the aging process. Foods that are rich in silica are rice, oats, lettuce, parsnips, asparagus, onion, strawberry, cabbage, cucumber, leek, sunflower seeds, celery, rhubarb, cauliflower, and Swiss chard.

Note that many of these foods, particularly rice, are a large part of Asian diets and Asians tend to have the strongest and healthiest hair. Be sure to seek out all the above foods from sources that grow food organically, as this is vital to obtaining the trace minerals that are usually not present in North American soil and therefore not in American foods. Additionally, these foods should be eaten uncooked, or in the case of rice-unwashed, as trace minerals are easily cooked and washed away.

Essential Fatty Acids (EFA's) are fatty acids needed by the body, yet not produced by the body. EFA's are a key component of healthy skin, hair, and nails. Common skin diseases, such as those discussed later in this book like eczema and seborrhea, are in part, caused by deficiencies in EFA's. Including deep-water fish such as salmon, sardines, mackerel, trout, or herring approximately three times, a week will provide sufficient amounts of EFA's. However, if the unable to eat deep-water fish or have an extreme dislike for it, it may be necessary to take a supplement to obtain the required amount of EFA's.

Finally, yet importantly, make sure to include the proper amount of water in your diet. **Water** is vital to proper hydration, which is necessary for all nutrients utilized properly by the body, not to mention the proper function of every cell in the body including hair follicles. The suggested amount of water intake daily is eight 8-ounce glasses of water a day, or 64 ounces a day.

The effects of high-fat diets and the increase of DHT (Dihydrotestosterone), a chemical produced by the body found to cause hair loss, is not conclusive at this time. However, there does seem to be a connection; as societies that consumed relatively low-fat diets such as pre-World War II Japan experienced almost no pattern baldness, whereas in post-World War II Japan there is an increase in pattern baldness as their society consumes a higher fat diet. In fact, Asian and African men in their native countries traditionally suffer very little Male Pattern Baldness (MPB).

Although when the same peoples come to North America, they begin to develop MPB. Because people of all races and ethnicities tend to develop MPB or androgenetic alopecia, yet do not exhibit these tendencies before moving to America, changes in diet may be a leading contributing factor. Diets high in fat do increase testosterone, which is the main component in DHT. To be conclusive, more research is needed, although it certainly could not hurt to lower one's fat intake.

Fiber is vital to making sure undigested food moves through the body and to the bowels properly. Failure of foods to move through the bowels in a reasonable amount of time can cause fermentation of undigested food in the bowels and block nutrients from being absorbed by the body. Beyond causing degrees of malnutrition, this can also cause a level of toxicity that will overwork systems in the body such as the adrenal glands and contribute to hair loss. Healthy amounts of fresh vegetables, fruits and legumes consumed daily will ensure a proper amount of dietary fiber.

If you feel it is unrealistic to eat properly due to your work schedule or dislike certain foods; then nutritional supplements containing these same vitamins and minerals are recommended. Be sure to take supplements naturally chelated, meaning, developed in a natural base. This will ensure that the supplements you consume will be more readily absorbed in the body. There are some cautions to taking supplements of certain vitamins and minerals, particularly those that are fat-soluble because the body stores them.

Vitamin A can be highly toxic, and supplements of vitamin A should be avoided unless recommended by a doctor. It is best to achieve one's vitamin A requirement either by food or through a naturally chelated multivitamin. Also, remember that smoking and second-hand smoke can cause blocking of vitamin A assimilation, so it is best to avoid smoking and remove one's self from areas and situations where second-hand smoke is present if possible.

Vitamin E supplements should always be taken at 400 i.u. per day to start and work your way up to 800 i.u. Always take vitamin E in its natural form, which is d-alpha tocopherol. Avoid taking vitamin E supplements in the synthetic form d-alpha tocopherol, derived from petroleum and is less available for assimilation into the body. If you have high blood pressure or other serious illnesses, consult a physician before taking vitamin E supplements.

Zinc is one fat-soluble mineral that can cause harm if an overdose occurs. Zinc can rob the body of copper, mentioned above as a key nutrient for hair growth and health, not to mention in other functions of the body. Zinc supplements should be taken in low doses, such as 5mg at a time. These are commonly be found in zinc lozenges designed for sore throats.

There is a "trick" to tell if you are taking too much zinc. When the zinc levels in the body surpassed the level that they can be absorbed, a metallic taste begins to form. If you pay attention to the metallic taste, you will know when enough zinc is in your body and stop taking it immediately.

You should not take iron supplements unless prescribed by your doctor for severe iron deficiency. If you do take an iron supplement, avoid ferrous sulfate, which you will find as the most common over-the-counter iron supplement in drug stores. Ferrous sulfate is hard for the body to assimilate, and because iron is not water-soluble, it will sit in the body and can cause severe liver problems over time.

Further, ferrous sulfate causes constipation, which can trigger a great deal more problems besides being extremely unpleasant. One iron supplement that does not contain ferrous sulfate is called Floradix and is available in both liquid and pill form.

Since there are so few foods to mention grown in North America that contain a good amount of silica, supplements may be needed. Nettle is also a good source of silica and Nettle Root Extract is readily available at health food stores.

Supplements of Essential Fatty Acids (EFA's) such as Evening Primrose Oil, Wheat Germ Oil, Flaxseed Oil, Cod Liver Oil, and other oils from deep-water fish are available at most grocery stores. It is not recommended to rely on Cod Liver Oil as a source for EFA's because it contains high levels of vitamins A and D, and the amount of Cod Liver Oil necessary to achieve proper amounts of EFA's would cause overdosing on these vitamins.

The recommended supplements are Evening Primrose Oil and Flaxseed Oil. Both these oils are available in oil form or capsules. Keep in mind that high amounts of the saturated fat block the effectiveness of EFA's, counteracting their effectiveness, so there need to be adjustments to your diet if there is a high amount of saturated fat in it.

Juicing is a natural way to obtain many of the vitamins, minerals, and trace minerals mentioned above. When using organic fruits and vegetables, juicing can provide quite a boost to the system and encourage the health of hair. The body very readily absorbs juices and provide the same content as the whole food. Fresh juices have a high enzyme content, which is beneficial to your body. Storing the juice or purchasing pasteurized juices from the store diminishes this benefit, although the benefits of the minerals and vitamins are usually still available.

You juice all of the fruits and vegetable mentioned to obtain the maximum benefit from them. A great deal of silica, sulfur, iron, and potassium, for example, is extracted from organic carrot juice. In fact, carrots being roots contain most trace minerals the body needs. You can enhance the effects of carrot juice by adding cucumber juice because of its high silica and sulfur content.

Organic spinach juice is highly recommended, as it is high in iron, vitamin A, and other vital vitamins and minerals; combined with lettuce and carrot juice, are two very good sources of silica and vitamin A. Unfortunately, you should avoid drinking non-organic spinach juice, which can be extremely high in pesticides. Do not take spinach juice if you suffer from kidney stones, as it contains a large amount of oxalic acid, shown in research studies to exacerbate kidney stone growth.

Other Hair Growth Foods

Looking for other foods that will help grow hair. Here is my recommended list of foods that promote hair growth:

- Essential fatty acids. Walnuts, canola oil, fish, and soy
- Iron rich foods. Liver, whole grain cereals, dark green leafy vegetables, eggs, and raisins

- Protein rich foods. Liver, brewer's yeast, fish, eggs, cottage cheese, and yogurt
- Vitamin D. Fortified orange juice
- Vitamin E. Avocados, nuts, seeds, and olive oil.

By contrast, hormone-regulating foods lack estrogen but work to stimulate your hormone production by adding nourishment to your endocrine glands. This creates a balance between your estrogen and testosterone levels, which affect hair loss, and growth. According to Dr. Gloria Chacon, hormone-regulating supplements "restore natural hormones in women, unlike hormone drugs, which override your body's natural endocrine functioning with synthetic hormones."

In the final chapter, I provide you with some motivation and inspiration to help build your confidence and to offer you a plan of action that you can use to chart your course toward feeling good about who you are and your contribution to the world. Yes, this book is about hair loss, it is also a book to give you hope and let you know that you are not alone. It is my hope that so far, the stories and advice I have given have given you the strength and courage to keep moving forward as we prepare to cross the finish line together. We are almost there.

Limit or Avoid these Foods

There are some foods and substances you should avoid or limit your consumption of them. Substances such as alcohol, caffeine, sugar and nicotine can deplete the body of nutrients and raise adrenal levels, which will cause a chain reaction of producing more androgen and causing hair loss. High levels of saturated fat and cholesterol rich foods are also linked to increased DHT levels, and their consumption should be limited.

In the next chapter, I compare Western (United States), and Eastern (Asian) approaches to dealing with nutrition and menopause.

Key Point#3

"The best way to maintain a healthy vitamin and mineral intake is a good diet."

5

East & West

While I have focused on women in the U.S, it is interesting to look at how women from Asia deal with menopause and hair loss. In the U.S., a woman has more emphasis placed on her beauty and hair. After menopause, many women will notice thinning scalp hair and increase in facial hair due to a drop in estrogen production.

After the onset of menopause, estrogens are no longer present, thereby exposing it to a similar although a milder type of syndrome that men experience with the overproduction of DHT. An interesting note is that the syndrome of menopause and its unique effects are not as common in the Eastern world, but are specific to Western civilization. The key differences are the consumption of less red meat and fatty foods in Eastern countries than in the West.

Another factor is the consumption of soybeans and soybean products is much higher in the East. This is significant because soy contains estrogens-like substances and work in the body similarly to estrogens. Therefore, there is not an extreme drop in estrogens levels in women who consume soybean products, thus reducing the symptoms of menopause typically suffered in the West.

Some women who suffer hair loss tend to have gastrointestinal problems that do not allow them to absorb proteins and zinc that are necessary to maintain a healthy head of hair. If you think that you have problems with your gastrointestinal system and are experiencing unusual hair loss, of course, see your doctor. You may be able to take some natural non-dairy acidophilus after meals for a couple of months in order to increase your digestion of these nutrients.

There are some myths associated with hair loss in women particularly. Many were told that brushing the hair 100 strokes each night would promote healthy hair growth. As mentioned earlier, extreme brushing of the hair can cause stress on the hair which can cause breakage and hair loss.

In addition, just as hats and wigs were rumored to cause hair loss, this is untrue; especially if the scalp is given sufficient time to breathe at night and hair is shampooed regularly to avoid buildup. [8]

Although stress can cause temporary hair loss, permanent hair loss is usually unconnected to stress. Finally, yet importantly, the belief that there are cosmetic products that are out on the market that grows hair is simply unfounded. There is only one FDA-approved product on the market that's proven to grow hair on women safely, and that is *Women's Rogaine®* I will address over the counter products later in the book.

In the upcoming chapter, I will discuss medical advances in identifying possible hormone causes of hair loss through blood screening tests. I have tried to balance the amount of information that is considered technical and medical without oversimplifying the issue. For those wishing to gain a deeper knowledge of blood testing techniques, I have added several footnotes with references to empirical research articles that you can read as a supplement to this book.

---

[8] Wearing hats and wigs too tight can cause constant traction or tightness, which can lead to hair loss called traction alopecia.

Key Point #4

"Menopause and its unique effects are not as common in the Eastern world... key differences are the consumption of less red meat and fatty foods."

6

It's in the Blood

It amazes me how important our blood system is in relation to prescribing treatment options. Today, we can find a wealth of information about a person, just from studying their blood. This is also true for studying your hair. When I review a client's blood work for analysis, I will explain to them how vitally important these blood tests are in helping to develop individualized treatment options. It is recommended that clients have their blood drawn by their primary physician following a 12 hour fast in the morning, preferably before breakfast and 10 a.m.

Blood tests are conducted by your physician as mention earlier, and sent to a lab for analysis, and recommended profile. Within a week or so, the results are sent to your physician, and in some cases, patients will bring their results to a Trichologist for analysis and explain how blood levels affect hair. Before I discuss reading a client's blood profile, it is important to understand several important hormones connected with hair loss.

Key Hormones Affecting Hair Loss

The role of hormones is to regulate cells and tissues activity in different organs of the body like your liver, heart, and skin. Hormones are secreted by your endocrine glands through the bloodstream, to tissues and organs where they affect body functions. A slight shift or imbalance of your hormones could lead to changes in your body as a whole. In most cases, hormonal issues are the general cause of hair loss. When your hormones are in balance with the rest of the body, you can enjoy good health and a feeling of well-being on the other hand, when your hormones are out of balance, you can feel sluggish, depressed, stressed and a host of other negative emotions.

Your most important sex hormones affecting hair loss are the following: *estrogens, progesterone, testosterone, cortisol,* and *Dehydroepiandrosterone.* Having a good understanding of these powerful hormones is vitally important to bringing your body into harmony and promoting good health.

Estrogens are responsible for stimulating tissue growth and the development of your breast and reproductive organs and makes sure they are functioning properly. In your brain, it acts as a booster for the synthesis of neurotransmitters, which affects sleep, memory, libido, mood, and cognitive function, which include your attention span and learning capabilities. It also acts to decreases your perception of pain, preserves bone mass, skin elasticity, and moisture; and increases the good cholesterol, HDL. Estrogens are essential to the dilation of your blood vessels and slows the formation of plague within your blood vessels as well.

The three major naturally occurring estrogens in women are estrone (E1), estradiol (E2) and estriol (E3). Estradiol is the predominate estrogen during reproductive years, both in terms of absolute serum levels as well as in terms of estrogenic activity.

Estradiol, which is the most potent, created by your ovaries, adrenals, and fat cells affect the majority of your body's organs. *Estriol*, the least active form of estrogen is primarily active during pregnancy. *Estrone* is produced mostly by your fatty cells and released into the body after menopause.

Progesterone promotes the development and function of your breasts and reproductive tract; made primarily by your ovaries, however; to a lesser degree, the adrenal glands, peripheral nerves, and brain cells produce it. Within your brain, it binds together various receptors that give you a sense of calm or sedating feeling; found to help with the quality of sleep and in preventing the onset of seizures.

Progesterone acts as a diuretic in eliminating excess water from the body, enhances your body's sensitivity to insulin and the activity of your thyroid hormones. Furthermore, it blocks plaque formation in your blood vessels, lowers triglycerides levels and strengthens your bones. It can also increase how your body burns fat as an efficient energy source.

Testosterone strengthens your bones, ligaments, and muscles; help promotes a sense of well-being and assertive behavior as well as your stamina sleep and helps to fights against cardiovascular disease.

The hormone, *dihydrotestosterone* or DHT is a potent form of testosterone. When you go through menopause, your estrogens levels decrease and is out of balance with DHT levels. High DHT can lead to genetic hair loss in women that are genetically predisposed to hair loss.

Dehydroepiandrosterone (DHEA). DHEA is an abundant circulating hormone, which protects you against the effective of inflammation in your body and negative physical stress. Similar to testosterone, it can increase sexual arousal, improve motivation, decreases pain, and improves your immune system functioning. Another powerful function of DHEA is its facilitation rapid eye movement (REM) phase of your sleep, improved memory, and maintenance of normal cholesterol levels. Your muscles, bones, and liver also converts DHEA into estrogens and testosterone.

Cortisol, produced by the adrenal glands regulates your immune response, stimulates glucose production, aids in short-term memory, and increases your body's heart rate, blood pressure, and respiration in response to stressful situations. Your level of cortisol is at its highest early in the morning when you are preparing to meet the demands of the day and gradually decreases until it reaches its lowest level late in the evening. This rise and fall of cortisol throughout the day is a pattern referred to as your body's "circadian rhythm."

Pregnenolone is the building block for all steroid hormones. Converted directly into DHEA and/or progesterone in the same way DHEA converts to testosterone and estrogens; and progesterone converts to cortisol, estrogen, and aldosterone. Pregnenolone is responsible for steroid hormone production in your body; created from cholesterol in the adrenal glands, liver, brain, skin, and retina of the eye. Similar to the hormones of estrogen and testosterone, pregnenolone can decrease with age. It is important to know that this repetitive cycle of succession and conversions are essential to making and sustaining human life.

Now that you have a better understanding of the functions of hormones in your body, I will discuss the use of blood tests in making a diagnosis and analysis of blood test profiles.

Profile Examination

A common profile examines your iron levels including ferritin, which I discussed earlier. In addition, white and red blood cells, zinc, vitamin B12, folic acid and thyroid panels are reviewed. Sometimes, hormonal and full blood chemistries are run. An Adrenal panel is run to rule out imbalances. It is important to understand, with hormone tests, they can be within normal ranges, and you still be affected with hair loss issues. Why is this?

A lot depends on your hair follicles sensitivity to circulating hormones in your blood. For example, if you are genetically predisposed to hair loss, then so-called normal levels of estrogens and androgens might create problems. It is also important to know that similar analysis of thyroid, iron, ferritin, B12, folic acid, that show in the normal ranges can also affect your hair follicles differently than in other people. Remember I said earlier that hair loss is personal; ranges are based on statistical models of the general population.

Below are some common blood tests and ranges:

Test	Levels
SHBG (Sex Hormone Binding Globulin):	Values around 90 are desirable. Values above 100 are considered too high.
Luteinizing Hormone (LH):	Normal levels: 5 to 20 IU/L
Luteinizing Hormone	Hormone: normal levels: 5 to 20 IU/L
Progesterone:	A value above 5 means a woman is ovulating. Progesterone: normal levels: Pre-ovulation: >1 ng/ml Midcycle: 5 to 20 ng/ml Postmenopausal: >1 ng/ml
Follicle Stimulating Hormone (FSH):	FSH: normal levels: Follicular: 3.5 to 12.5 IU/L Midcycle: 4.7 to 21.5 IU/L Postmenopausal: 25.8 to 134.8 IU/L
DHEA and DHEAS	DHEA: normal level for women by age: 18 to 29 years: 62 to 615 ug/dL 30 to 39 years: 52 to 400 ug/dL 40 to 49 years: 44 to 352 ug/dL 50 to 59 years: 39 to 183 ug/dL 60+ years: 11 to 150 ug/dL
Adrenal Panel:	Done to rule out adrenal deficiencies
Estradiol:	Normal levels: premenopausal: 20 to 400 pg/ml Postmenopausal: 5 to 25 pg/ml
Testosterone:	normal levels: 20 to 80 ng/dl
T3 and T4:	Best TSH value is between 1 and 2. Values above 3 are still considered normal by many labs (the upper level of normal is 5) usually indicates an overactive thyroid
TSH (Thyroid Stimulating Hormone):	Optimum level: .3 to 3.0 mlU/L if you are on thyroid medication, between .5 and 2.0 mlU/L

Reading Blood Test Results

As a case study, let us suppose you had blood drawn and waited for your results, you schedule a meeting with your doctor, then during your visit, she pulls up your blood work and says, "Everything looks good, and your numbers are within their normal ranges." Remember, ranges are based on a statistical distribution of the general population. Chances are good you might be wondering, "Did the doctor miss something?" You are still worried because you know something is going on in your body causing your hair to thin, recede, or fall out in clumps.

Perhaps, the problem is how your doctor may interpret the lab results. Your doctor may be looking for levels that will negatively influence your overall general health. However, a Trichologist recognizes different levels of normal. As an example, there could be *low normal, mid-normal and high normal* ranges.

As a Trichologist, I understand that high and low normal ranges could affect your hair and not your overall health from a physiology viewpoint. This would be the case for ferritin with a reference range of 10-130 ug/L (micrograms per litre), with your results showing a reading of 30 ug/L. To your doctor, this would be okay with respect to your general health, however, for hair, the optimum level should be at least 80 ug/L. less than that could increase chances of hair loss or decrease your hair growth.

Other hormone range readings can also show normal, but affect your hair growth, such as Thyroid and hemoglobin levels, which are complex. Here is my advice, after you have spoken with your physician about hair loss, and you still have concerns; schedule a meeting with a certified Trichologist to review your blood work and offer further analysis and treatment options.

Key Point #5

"After you have spoken with your physician about hair loss, and you still have concerns; have a certified Trichologist review your blood work to offer analysis and treatment options."

7

What About Other Options?

To be balanced and fair, there is a lot of talk about over-the-counter products and prescription medications proven to help regrow hair. I feel it is important to address some of these options.

In this chapter, I will discuss five common products on the market for re-growing hair. These are Rogaine®, Propecia® Aldactone, Zinc Pyrithione ZnP, and Betamethasone valerate.

The most popular over-the-counter hair restoration treatment today is Rogaine®, a topical minoxidil solution developed by the Pfizer Corporation and approved for over the counter sale in by the Food and Drug Administration (FDA) in 1997. Did you know that its key ingredient, Minoxidil was originally used as a blood pressure medication? Then, by accident, doctors found that it produced as a side effect increased scalp hair growth.

Minoxidil remains the only FDA approved pharmaceutical topical solution proven to grow hair. In preliminary studies held in 1985, about 55% of men tested re-grew hair with extra strength Rogaine® (5% topical minoxidil treatment), The best results came from those who had been balding less than 10 years and were bald in a section of four inches across or less.

In another test, which compared the results of regular strength Rogaine® (2% topical minoxidil solution) with the extra strength version, found that those tested, grew 45% more hair with the extra strength Rogaine® than with the regular strength Rogaine®, and users of both solutions outgrew the users of the placebo.[9]

Only 6% of those tested experienced any type of irritation. Rogaine® works by blocking the production of DHT, which I have discussed previously. Rogaine® was originally made only for men's use, and then a women's version of the drug was produced with similar results, it should be noted that

[9] https://www.ncbi.nlm.nih.gov/pubmed/12196747

both versions continuous use of the drug is necessary to maintain the newly grown hair, as it is a usual reaction for newly growing hair to stop growing and fall out when you cease to use the drug. As with any drug, follow all directions and cease to use if irritation or discomfort persists. [10]

A popular prescription drug treatment which can be prescribed by your doctor is Propecia® brand Finasteride created by Merck & Company, Inc. It is the only FDA-approved pill approved for the prevention of hair loss and possible hair re-growth. Like Rogaine®, Propecia® discovered when its generic equivalent being used for another purpose, also showed beneficial side effects.

Finasteride is the generic name for the drug, which was already in existence for quite some time and produced under the name Proscar® by Merck & Company and used for the treatment of enlarged prostates, a syndrome medically called benign prostatic hyperplasia (BPH). BPH is caused by an overproduction of DHT, which causes the prostate to grow.

Many BHP patients were also suffering from baldness, and when patients began taking Proscar®, they noticed the re-growth of hair. This sparked new testing and the birth of Propecia® as a hair restoration drug, easily approved by the

---

[10] https://clinicaltrials.gov/ct2/show/NCT01145625

FDA since it was merely marketing already approved Finasteride as a hair restoration drug, with a much smaller dosage than required for BPH, which is an androgen hormone inhibitor. There are research studies that show Finasteride could be effective in post-menopausal women, as one double-blind research study showed, "successful treatment was subsequently reported in post-menopausal women, albeit sometimes with higher doses over longer treatment periods.

A 67-year-old woman with an history of progressive hair thinning and no laboratory evidence of hyperandrogenism was unable to tolerate antiandrogen therapy with spironolactone 100 mg/d, and a switch to cyproterone 50 mg was ineffective.

Finasteride 5 mg once weekly was started, and after 12 months the patient reported increased hair density and standardized global photography of her scalp showed significant hair regrowth." [11]

Unfortunately, the drug is not approved for use by women at this time, especially women who are pregnant or can become pregnant, because the conversion of testosterone to DHT can affect secondary sex characteristics of unborn fetuses. It can,

[11] http://www.dpic.org/article/professional/finasteride-hair-loss-women.

however, be prescribed as an 'off -label' prescription by a doctor since they can legally prescribe any medication(s) they deem appropriate for treatment.

Propecia® works by reducing DHT production. It works best in combination with topical treatments of Minoxidil such as Rogaine®. Participants in research studies have seen hair growth in as little as six months, whereas those who have seen no results in a year's time are reported not likely to see any results from the drug.

Aldactone is the brand prescription medication for spironolactone, used in pill form to treat three common issues: acne, hirsutism (too much hair on the face), and androgenetic alopecia. According to the *British Journal of Dermatology* (2005), eighty percent of women receiving oral spironolactone could expect to see a cessation their female pattern hair loss, with an improved chance of re-growing hair after taking 200 milligrams a day for a year.

Zinc Pyrithione ZnP solution has been shown to kill bacteria and yeast in the oil glands and hair follicles which can lead to healthier hair. [12] It also may inhibit 5-alpha-reductase in the hair follicle. When used by post-menopausal women in one research study, it resulted in thicker hair after twelve months

---

[12] https://www.ncbi.nlm.nih.gov/pubmed/21272039

of use. Researchers are unsure why it works. Other topical medications used as a topical scalp lotion to block androgen receptor sites include progesterone, zinc salts, azelaic acid, flutamide, dutasteride, and finasteride.[13]

Betamethasone valerate (cortisone) in another research study indicated that when used daily as a topical solution for a year led to thicker hair. Many doctors who specialize in hair loss make up their own prescription blend of a few or most of the medications listed above.[14]

Alternative Recommendations

I realize that many of you may not choose to use over-the - counter or prescription medications to treat your hair loss condition in order avoid chemicals and their possible side effects. The first level of treatment are herbal remedies combined with scalp massages to stimulate hair follicles and help your hair to regenerate. Herbal remedies are the only viable option to dealing with a hormonal imbalance at its source, which involves eating *phytoestrogen* foods discussed in chapter 7.

In my professional opinion, Nettle Root Extract and Sal Palmetto has been an effective herbal treatment in blocking

---

[13] http://www.science.gov/topicpages/z/zinc+pyrithione+shampoo.html
[14] https://www.ncbi.nlm.nih.gov/pmc/articles/PMC3149478/

the production of DHT and work similar to topical Minoxidil products. I feel that it is my duty to provide you with a range of options so you can make an informed and balanced decision for yourself.

In the next chapter, I discuss how eating twelve powerful foods can help improve hair growth and slow the hair loss process.

Key Point #6

"Nettle Root Extract has been an effective herbal treatment in blocking the production of DHT and work similar to topical Minoxidil products."

8

Power of Twelve

If you recall back in Chapter 3, I discussed at length the role vitamins and minerals play in the maintenance, growth, and restoration of hair in women. In this chapter, we look at twelve power foods shown to be rich in *phytoestrogens,* and importance of making them a part of your hormone balanced diet.

What are Phytoestrogenic Foods?

Phytoestrogenic foods are foods that contain estrogenic components produced by plants, which can help, bring your estrogen levels in balance with the rest of your body's system. For example, 100g of vegetables such as broccoli, green beans, winter squash and garlic contain between 94 to 604mcg of phytoestrogens.

As a word of caution, these foods will at first treat hormonal imbalances, but long-term use of plant-based estrogens into your body could cause your body to stop producing its own estrogen resulting in further decreased estrogen levels. Besides the consumption of estrogen rich foods, avoid or reduce your alcohol intake. Also, include stress reduction exercises such as Tai chi, meditation, and yoga into your daily regimen. As a side note, you should avoid eating these foods if your estrogen levels are too high.

Here are twelve foods that help produce hair growth.

1. *Alfalfa Sprouts*

Alfalfa sprouts are low in calories, carbohydrates and contain phytonutrients and plant estrogen, which lacks the side effects, associated with other forms of estrogen supplementation and is a good vegetable to eat in the on salads, and sandwiches.

2. *Beans*

It is no secret that beans are high in fiber and have the ability to lower bad cholesterol, what is seldom known about beans is they also contain phytoestrogens. Beans are the major substitute for meat because of their protein content, and will fill you up quickly and digest slowly; a great choice for those who are diabetic or those who need to maintain balanced glucose levels. Bean are often eaten as a side dish, and most families use beans as a staple food for a number of dishes.

4. *Bran Cereals*

Bran is best known as being high in fiber and several years ago food such as bran muffins and fiber cereals like as All-Bran and Fiber One, were very popular. Wheat fiber is also a source of phytoestrogens

5. *Chickpeas*

Chickpeas commonly eaten as a form of hummus or falafel, and because they lack flavor, they can be mixed with other foods, spices, and seasonings. Also, a *phytoestrogen*, they are high in fiber and protein, an alternative to meat consumption.

6. *Dried Fruits*

Dried fruits like apricots, dates, and prunes, help to balance your estrogen levels and add fiber to your diet because they contain *phytoestrogens*, which mimics how your body uses estrogen by restoring any estrogen shortages and it produces the similar effect as real estrogen in your body. Another factor that helps is the higher concentration of phytoestrogens due to the dying process itself.

One drawback is that the drying process also concentrates higher sugar levels, so you don't need to eat as much as you would fresh fruit to the same effect. They are best eaten during the spring months. 100g dried dates contain 330mcg of phytoestrogens, while dried apricots contain 445 mcg. Other fruits like raspberries, strawberries, and peaches, contain 48 to 65mcg per 100g serving.

7. *Flaxseeds*

Most people will eat flaxseeds on their salads, and others prefer to eat them directly. For example, ground flaxseed when used in cooking will disappear in smoothies or soups. Because they are high in fiber, they will speed up a sluggish digestive system. Another great benefit is that they can lower your cholesterol levels. Flaxseeds also have omega-3s that will keep your arteries from hardening, a major cause of strokes and heart attacks.

8. *Peas*

Peas, mainly eaten as a side dish or in casseroles and offer a number of minerals like magnesium, iron, and potassium, and some protein, as well as phytoestrogens; they are also a source of Vitamin C, which can boost your immune system.

Overall, you will be healthier with fewer symptoms connected to menopause and post-menopause by eating peas.

9. *Sesame Seeds*

Sesame seeds contain lignin, which possesses phytoestrogens. Like Dried fruits and flaxseeds, they are high in fiber; one tablespoon gives you about 4 % of your daily allowance of fiber and minerals such as iron, calcium, and magnesium. Due to size, you can incorporate them easily into your meals or use them to make the crust.

10. *Soybeans*

In a way, soybeans are considered a super food since other foods derive from soybeans such as tofu, tempeh, and soymilk. Soybeans are extremely high in fiber and protein, and minerals like iron, magnesium, calcium and potassium. Soybeans can be cooked and added to salads or eaten as edamame, a raw form of soybean used as a snack or appetizer. By not having a strong flavor, it's easy for soybeans to get absorbed into surrounding flavors.

11. *Soy Milk*

Soy Milk is another food derived from soy provides the same benefits as tofu, tempeh, and soybeans in regards to phytoestrogens. In milk form, it easily enters the body and is quickly absorbed, increasing your estrogen levels. It will also curb a few symptoms associated with post-menopause by restoring some of the estrogens with phytoestrogens. Like milk, it is a great source of calcium, and for many, it is an alternative to drinking cow's milk.

12. *Tofu*

Tofu is food that is rich in isoflavones, which interact with your estrogen receptors. Tofu, contain *genistein*, which mimics the effects of estrogen. In large quantities, these may lessen menopausal symptoms. Tofu is also a great meat alternative for vegans and vegetarians because of its protein and iron content.

Tofu is preferred as a meat alternative because you get the good nutrients and avoid some of the bad properties associated with eating certain types of meats. It is recommended that you designate one or two days a week as meatless days by using tofu as meat substitutes in your meals; it will also give you more estrogen than eating beef or chicken.

In the final chapter, I provide you with some motivation and inspiration to help build your confidence and to offer you a plan of action that you can use to chart your course toward feeling good about who you are and your contribution to the world. Yes, this book is about hair loss, it is also a book to give you hope and let you know that you are not alone. It is my hope that so far, the stories and advice I have given have given you the strength and courage to keep moving forward as we prepare to cross the finish line together. We are almost there.

Key Point #7

"Phytoestrogenic foods contain estrogenic components which can help bring your estrogen levels in balance with the rest of your body's system."

9

Why Seek Inspiration?

In this chapter, I discuss the importance of inspiration. As I mentioned before, this book has three main purposes, first, to provide information on the causes of hair loss due to menopause. Second, to recommend holistic treatment options proven to regrow hair. The third and final purpose of this book is to help you regain your confidence by providing you with words of inspiration and motivation that you can recite as personal affirmations or read as part of your daily devotion.

It is my strongest belief that without a positive vision of the future, you may fall victim to the negative forces that exist in the world. These negative forces are not some scary shadows; they are the negative self-talk we tell ourselves that things are not going to get better. I refuse to accept that line of thinking, as long as you have breath in your body; you can change how you feel and see yourself. It begins with you.

In this chapter, I will shift gears to talk about the importance of seeking out things and people who inspire you to keep moving forward. For anything excellent and great that you wish to accomplish in your life, there's one imperative requirement - inspiration. This is true as you deal with your hair loss. A great inspiration brings with it a wave of power that by itself may propel you over the finish line. Conversely, when we are empty of inspiration, everything may appear hard, boring and dull, and we acquire no joy out of what we're doing.

Inspiration is crucial as it keeps the mind positive and centered on the greater picture, when we fail to do this, our thoughts can act as a barrier to our self-growth.

The mind is prone to wavering and doubt, shifting from one way to the other at a moment's notice. Frequently when you feel a deep inner yearning to achieve something, the mind will initially go along with it, lured by the novelty factor. Nevertheless, when the going gets fierce, and you start to encounter roadblocks in accomplishing your goal, the mind will frequently be the first one to jump ship! By bringing in outer sources of inspiration to your life, you help your mind "see the forest for the trees" and work with you to accomplish your goals.

Occasionally the process of bringing purpose and meaning of your life means you have to boldly step into territory unmapped by most of the individuals around you. You start to explore choices beyond the nine-to-five cycle of eating, working and sleeping, and start to move away towards a deeper sense of being.

As many of those around you aren't as interested as you are in living out your total potential, it's simple to feel that you're plowing a lone furrow, and this may make you question if indeed you're doing the right thing. That's why staying in touch with inspiring individuals and reading inspiring stories is so crucial, as it lets, you see that other people have been in the same place as you.

That is why I added the case studies of Maggie and Jill, to let you know you are not alone in this journey. If they have gone on to accomplish their goal of regaining their hair and confidence, then why can't you? As the mind gets bored of new things quickly, you perpetually need to refill your source of inspiration:

Having like-minded individuals around you can be excellent in that regard - you can guarantee that if one individual in the group isn't feeling particularly inspired, somebody else will be, and their inspiration will act as a lift-me-up tonic. I created a Face Book group where you can share your stories, ideas and offer support to other women. Likewise, together we serve as a valuable source of fresh ideas - when one individual discovers something that works for them, and then he or she may share that with everybody else.

Reading may be a powerful source of inspiration, as it directly bears upon the mind. Reading personal inspirational stories may be particularly powerful, as you are able to put yourself in the shoes of that individual and imagine yourself overcoming those roadblocks.

You can utilize the inspiration you have as a launching pad to increase your desires - you're inner yearning for fulfillment. Many individuals who give seminars on success in different areas all state the same thing - that the difference between accomplishing a goal and not accomplishing it is merely whether how much you desired it.

The very act of increasing your desire to overcome obstacles helps to move you away from negative feelings and situations and to bring about the changes you wish to see in your life. In the next chapter I share four of my favorite recipes are (1) Sesame chicken pasta salad, (2) Asparagus with lemon-garlic sauce, (3) Grilled chicken with fresh spring mix and warmed chickpeas salad, and Rhubarbs Crumbles.

10

Estrogen Rich Recipes

Sesame Chicken Pasta Salad
By Chef Michael Porter

Ingredients needed:

1/4 cup sesame seeds

1 (16 ounce) package bow tie pasta

1/2 cup vegetable oil

1/3 cup light soy sauce

1 teaspoon sesame oil

2 tablespoons white sugar

1/2 teaspoon ground ginger

1/4 teaspoon ground black pepper

3 cups shredded, cooked chicken breast meat

1/3 cup chopped fresh cilantro

1/3 cup chopped green onion

1/3 cups shredded carrots

1/3 cups snap peas

Preparation:

Heat a skillet over medium-high heat. Add sesame seeds, and cook stirring frequently until lightly toasted.
Remove from heat, and set aside.

Bring a large pot of lightly salted water to a boil. Add pasta, and cook for 8 to 10 minutes, or until al dente. Drain pasta, and rinse under cold water until cool. Transfer to a large bowl.

In a jar with a tight lid, combine vegetable oil, soy sauce, sesame oil, sugar, sesame seeds, ginger, and pepper. Shake well.

Pour sesame dressing over pasta, and toss to coat evenly. Gently mix in chicken, cilantro, and green onions, shredded carrots, and snap peas.

Grilled Chicken with Fresh Spring Mix and Warmed Chick Peas Salad
By Chef Michael Porter

Ingredients needed:

6 tablespoons olive oil, plus more for drizzling

1 can chickpeas, rinsed

2 sprigs thyme

¼ teaspoon crushed red pepper flakes

4 small boneless skinless chicken breast (about 2½ lb. total)

Kosher salt and freshly ground black pepper

3 cups spring mix salad

2 tablespoon finely grated lemon zest

2 tablespoons fresh lemon juice

Preparation

Heat 2 Tbsp. oil in a medium skillet over medium-high heat; cook chickpeas, thyme, and red pepper flakes, stirring occasionally, just until warmed through, about 5 minutes. Transfer to a large bowl.

Prepare a grill for medium heat; oil grill grate. Brush chicken with 4 Tbsp. oil; season with salt and pepper. Grill chicken, skin side down, until golden brown and lightly charred, 8–10 minutes. Turn and grill until cooked through, 4 minutes longer.

Toss spring mix, lemon zest, and lemon juice into chickpeas. Serve with chicken, drizzled with more oil and sprinkled with sea salt.

Asparagus with Lemon-Garlic Sauce
By Chef Jay Jones

Ingredients needed:

3 cloves garlic diced softly

1/3 cake silken tofu

3 T. lemon juice

1/4 c. chopped scallion

Sea salt to liking

1 pound fresh asparagus

Preparation:

Mince the garlic. Blend the tofu, lemon juice, scallion and garlic in a food processor until smooth. Salt to taste. Add a little more lemon if needed. Steam the asparagus for 3 to 4 minutes until bright green. On med heat then place it on a plate and cover with sauce.

Serving Size 4. (One half portion soy per serving.)

Rhubarbs Crumbles
by Chef Michael Porter

TOPPING:

1/4 c chopped walnuts

2/4 c flax seed

1/3 c maple syrup

1 1/2 t. vanilla extract

FILLING:

1 c frozen apple juice concentrate

1/4 c cornstarch

6 c sliced rhubarb

1/4 c maple syrup

Preparation:

Preheat the oven to 300 or 320 degrees. To prepare topping, grind flaxseed in a manual grinder or electric coffee grinder. Place it in a mixing bowl. Add the nuts, maple syrup & vanilla & mix thoroughly. Spread the mixture on a cookie sheet or a non-stick baking pan & bake for 5 minutes, until toasted to your liking.

To prepare the filling, place a juice concentrate in a heavy bottomed saucepan. Add the rhubarb. Cook over medium heat until the rhubarb is soft (10 to 15 minutes). Dissolve the cornstarch in the maple syrup. Stir this into the rhubarb and stir continuously until the mixture thickens. Remove from heat. Pour into a 9-inch pie plate. Spoon the crumble over the fruit. Serve warm or cold.

Serving Size: 6. (2 portions per stir.

My Final Thoughts

As I prepare to end this chapter, I felt it important to express my sincere thanks and gratitude for purchasing this book. It is my deepest desire that this book has answered your questions about hair loss, offered you alternative yet, effective solutions that you can apply in place of using harsh chemicals, which can damage your hair. More important, I hope that this chapter has given you the strength to press on and never give up.

Printed in Great Britain
by Amazon